W9-CGT-907

BABY'S FIRST
100 DAYS

BABY'S FIRST
100 DAYS

Margaret Stephenson Meere,
BA, BHSc, RN, RM

BONNEVILLE BOOKS
SPRINGVILLE, UTAH

© 2011 Margaret Stephenson Meere
All rights reserved.
Author and text photos by Louise Lister Photography

No part of this book may be reproduced in any form whatsoever, whether by graphic, visual, electronic, film, microfilm, tape recording, or any other means, without prior written permission of the publisher, except in the case of brief passages embodied in critical reviews and articles.

The information provided in this book is intended for general information and guidance only, and should not be used as a substitute for consulting a qualified health practitioner. Neither the author nor the publisher can accept responsibility for any problems arising out of the contents of this book.

ISBN 13: 978-1-59955-917-9

Published by Bonneville Books, an imprint of Cedar Fort, Inc.,
2373 W. 700 S., Springville, UT 84663
Distributed by Cedar Fort, Inc., www.cedarfort.com

First published in 2001 in Australia and New Zealand by Doubleday.
The author and publishers are grateful to Tweddle Child and Family Services for permission to include a sleep cycle graph similar to that which appears in *Sleep Right Sleep Tight: a practical proven guide to solving your baby's sleep problems.*

Cover design by Megan Whittier
Cover design © 2011 by Lyle Mortimer
Edited and typeset by Melissa J. Caldwell

Printed in the United States of America
10 9 8 7 6 5 4 3 2 1
Printed on acid-free paper

*This book is dedicated to
my children—Richard,
Matthew, James, and David.*

CONTENTS

� · ✄ · ✄

CONTENTS

CONTENTS

ACKNOWLEDGMENTS

I have been blessed, in my life, with great teachers. To all the babies who brought their wonderful parents into my life—thank you. Especially Amelia and Susan, who started me thinking about the nature of crying, and Jordan, who taught me more about the pacifier than I realized at the time. Thanks also to Alexis, who brought Jenny Cooke along to guide (or goad) me into publication—I needed that push!

I owe a lot to my nursing colleagues, particularly to Fram Robinson, who trusted me enough to allow me creative freedom, and to Lesley Shanley and Cathie O'Brien, who supported me in the creative process.

The organizers and facilitators of People Know-how (now Zoeros) pointed the way to a less-traveled path, which I chose to tread and continue to follow.

Richard, Matthew, James, and David, who paid me the highest compliment in choosing me to be their mother, have given me more than thirty years of happiness, frustration, and fun. My appreciation, love, and admiration for them are immeasurable.

And, of course, to Midge, Ione, Fin, and Zeph, who keep me on my toes in the Grandma department, I give my grateful thanks.

❀ • ❀ • ❀ • ❀ • ❀

"It's not fair. You always experiment with me."
—*Richard, age 9, the eldest.*

Richard, you were so right.

❀ • ❀ • ❀ • ❀ • ❀

All babies are stars. Thank you Kate Noack, Alexandra Hofman, and Jackson Price, who are pictured in this book.

INTRODUCTION

This is a book of parenting that places less emphasis on scientific reasoning and offers some commonsense suggestions so that you can relate to it, and come to your own understanding of what is natural newborn baby behavior. You may then find it easier to make your own decisions about parenting the little person in your care.

If you have just had a new baby, then chances are that you are on the biggest learning curve of your life.

If you are a new grandparent, then you are on a pretty big learning curve as well. Part of this learning is about accepting that things are a little bit different from when you were a new parent.

Parenting a new parent is about being supportive

when needed. It's learning alongside the new parent and holding back on giving advice unless it is asked for; it's offering your shoulder for crying on, sharing the joy of new life, and settling back and enjoying a true experience of unconditional love. Appreciate the truth and humor of a bumper sticker that said simply:

"If I'd known being a grandparent was so much fun, I'd have done it first."

If you are the friend of a new parent, then share the opportunity of loving and learning—you'll be a whiz when it's your turn!

If you are a health professional, then I hope this way of looking at a continuum complements the wealth of knowledge that you already have.

The information in this book is just that—information. There is a ton of it around these days. The information here is not a collection of "musts" and "shoulds." It is something to think about, to use if you like it, and to add to other information. What appears on the following pages grew out of years of learning and observation, and most important, of listening to babies and their parents, particularly my own.

I hope you enjoy it and that it helps!

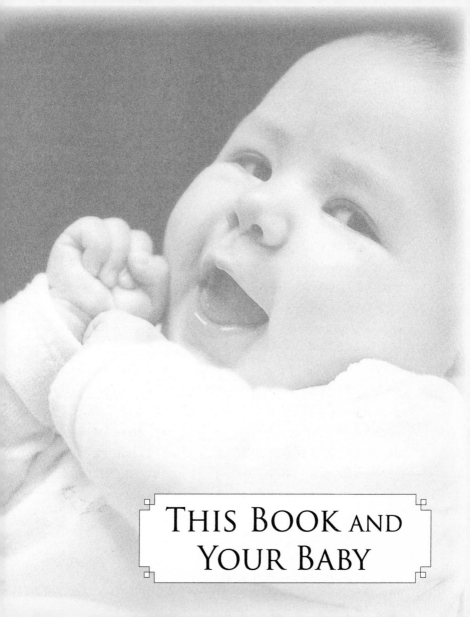

This Book and Your Baby

This book, like some babies, was unplanned.

It was conceived on an answering machine after a long weekend.

It had its gestation in the development of a teaching session I offered to new parents so that the questions that they so frequently asked by phone or in consultation could be answered in one go. Often these sessions were lively and very educational, not only for the parents and grandparents who attended, but also for my colleagues and me. We were all able to learn from each other, bounce ideas around, and have a good laugh.

Then the telephone quieted down.

The book is born to a wider participation and it goes with a hope that it too can generate some lively discussion sessions within families and parent groups. Its main purpose is to normalize a confusing period of a baby's life as early as possible. It can also be a source of reference for some of your questions.

It amazes me that as humans we can bring home a kitten, puppy, or other baby creature and nurture it with a sense of fun and confidence, and yet when we bring home our own human baby, we fret and lose our confidence.

Parenting can be fun—let's go and create it!

THE "AVERAGE" BABY

Now this is a tricky one.

Out there in the big wide world, a genius is born every few days, and he or she always upsets the "average" theory and therefore the contents of this book.

These little geniuses hardly ever cry. They burp on cue, fart discreetly, and smile the moment they are born.

However, it needs to be pointed out that the baby in this book is the average baby, and most of you will have one in at least one or more of the following chapters.

The "average" baby is either a boy or a girl, so in the following chapters, the baby is either a "he" or "she" but never a "he/she," which is politically correct but reduces the baby to somewhere in the middle. Just because the baby in the chapter on crying is a "she" and the baby in the chapter on sleeping is a "he" does not mean that girls cry more than boys and that boys sleep more than girls. It just makes for easier reading.

THE AGE OF A BABY

There are ages defined in terms of days, weeks, months, and years. The age of a baby is generally calculated in days during the first 1–2 weeks, and then in weeks during the first 3–4 months because a week at this stage of the baby's behavioral development is a long time.

After these 100 days or 14 weeks, a baby's age can be calculated in months using the baby's birth date.

That is, if baby is born on January 14, then she is 4 months of age on May 14.

When considering the development of a new baby's behavior during these first 100 days, it is important to consider whether the baby was born earlier or later than her expected date of birth.

If she was born a week or more early, then she may take a little longer to develop into the phases as described in the following chapters. If she was born

1–2 weeks later, then she may come earlier to these phases.

A "term" baby is a baby who is born after 37 weeks of pregnancy.

A "newborn" baby is a baby in her first month of life. After her first month, she is an infant until she is 12 months old.

In this book, the baby is a "new baby" for her first 100 days, and a "newborn" baby if the information is specific to her first month.

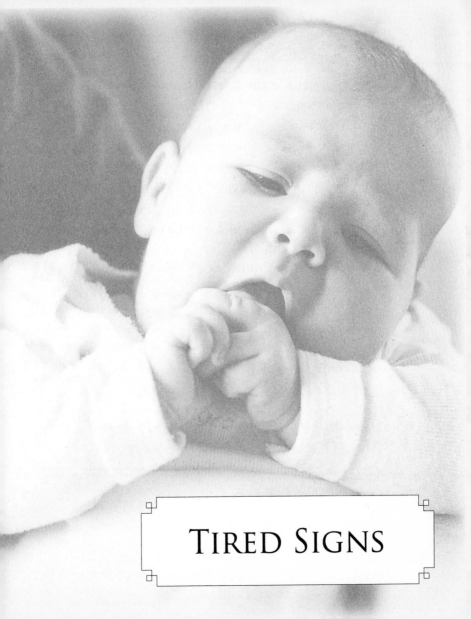

TIRED SIGNS

When a baby is tired, he gives us definite signs, but often we confuse them with hunger because there is a lot of mouth action and often a bit of noise. We can also confuse tired signs with what we think is pain or "colic" because baby will often draw his legs up in an effort to get himself into the fetal position, or he may go rigid like a banana. So here are some clues to tired signs in a new baby.

Frowning: one minute, baby appears content, then he loses eye contact with you and looks away. There may be a definite frown over the forehead and eyes.

Clenched fists: baby's hands are no longer open and relaxed but are tightly closed.

Hand-to-mouth action: this is fairly haphazard and he can end up scratching his cheek or eyes, when what he is attempting to do is suck on a finger or thumb in order to comfort himself.

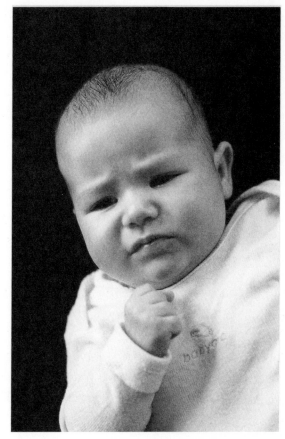

Frowning and clenched fists

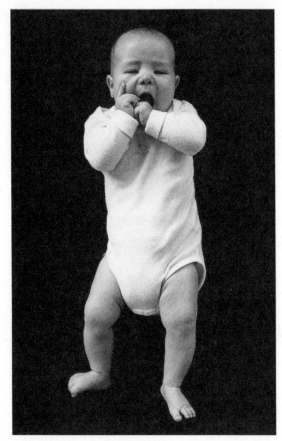

Hand-to-mouth action

Jerky movements: particularly with his arms.

Yawning: the best tired sign for the rest of his life. If you are around to see baby yawn, put him to bed now.

Grizzling: this starts out on a low scale and then proceeds to full on crying. However, this cry is very guttural, like a growl.

The body becomes tense as it becomes tired. When we are tired, our breathing becomes shallow, and the oxygen intake is low so the body responds by yawning to boost the oxygen level. Shallow breathing is the result of a tight diaphragm, tense muscles, high shoulders, and an anxious tummy.

If the tired signs are ignored—or if distraction is used to try to stop them—then it becomes much more difficult to settle the baby.

The more we handle him, the louder and more desperate he becomes.

Red in the face, body unrelaxed and stiff, baby ends up being rocked frantically, having a toy jangled in his face, or being passed from one person to the next.

He won't like it!

Baby needs to go to his bed to settle and sleep as soon as he gives you his tired sign. No delay.

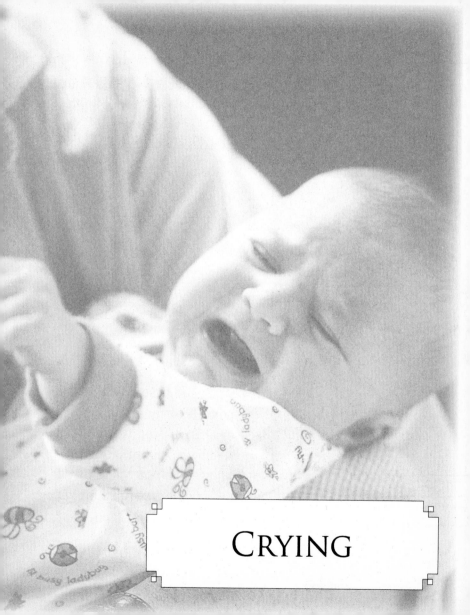

CRYING

Crying is a natural event. A new baby cries on average 2½ hours a day, and if nearly all babies do it, then there is a positive reason for this. The negative experience is for anyone who is around to hear it.

THE POSITIVES OF CRYING

- Watch your baby next time she is crying, and you will see some very good physical activity. Consider that crying, for a new baby, is not an emotional experience; it is a physical one.

- Crying is the only time that a new baby gets to fully expand her lungs so that they can develop and become healthy. If you observe your baby when she is deeply asleep, it is almost impossible to see her breathing because it is so shallow. The body is resting, there is no exercise, and her full lung capacity is not being used.

- Crying is the only way that a baby can un-
  wind and blow off the excess energy and
  excitement that has built up during her
  "awake" period. Older infants, children,
  and adults can do this by talking and running around.

---

*Hold your hand very close to your mouth as
you exhale strongly and feel the warmth. This
spent energy comes with your breath.*

HOW MUCH CRYING?

- From about 2–9 weeks of age, expect 1 unsettled period in a day and 1 unsettled day
  in a week. This 7-week period can be a tiring time for you and baby.

- The unsettled period can extend between

two feedings, when baby will be wakeful and/or crying and may only sleep fitfully. Often this period is in the evening when you are tired, when the milk supply may be running a little low, and when you are also trying to prepare and eat your own meal. It may make it easier to tolerate if you imagine that there are only about 49 of these unsettled periods (7 days x 7 weeks).

- The unsettled day or baby's "bad hair day" often occurs on a Sunday or Monday, because a baby is handled a lot more on weekends—in and out of the car seat, the stroller, and her bed, and out visiting, having visitors, and so on. Imagine that there will be about 7 unsettled days.

- Baby may cry about 30 minutes to 1 hour after the end of a feed because she is tired. There are scientific theories that suggest that when food reaches upper sections of the gut, a message is relayed to the brain that says, "sleep." This might explain why we feel so sleepy after eating a heavy meal, such as Christmas dinner.

- The time that a new baby spends crying generally peaks at about 6 weeks of age. From then on she will spend less time crying and more time awake during the daytime as she becomes a more social little person and begins to smile and vocalize in response to you.

- A baby's crying is most desperate when she is overtired. When a baby cries with such intensity, her little face will become very red and sweaty, and she will reach a stage of almost holding her breath. This is also quite distressing for anyone who can hear her, but often if a baby is able to move through this frenzy, she will fall asleep and sleep very well. This is because when a baby cries like this, she hyperventilates and breathes out too much carbon dioxide. The brief holding of breath stops this process, so the body feels more comfortable, the baby relaxes, and is able to put herself to sleep.

TYPES OF CRYING

At first, understanding the crying baby can be confusing, particularly with a new baby whom you are only beginning to get to know.

Hurting cry. If you were around to hear your baby cry when she had her heel pricked for her newborn screening test, you would have heard her scream with a high-pitched cry. That is her cry of pain.

Hunger cry. This is the cry that comes around three or four hours after the beginning of her last feed. It is a medium-pitched and medium intensity cry.

Tired cry. This commences with grizzling or grunting and can develop into a deep growl. It is quite guttural and may accompany a lot of hand-to-mouth action and stiffening or arching of the body.

"Something wrong" cry. This can be a concern and even difficult to define. If you feel intuitively that there is something wrong with your baby and you have ruled out tiredness or hunger, then seek medical advice as soon as possible. If you are not getting an answer that you feel comfortable with, then seek a second opinion.

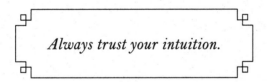

Always trust your intuition.

Does a baby have a "wet diaper cry"? Generally, a baby is only uncomfortable with a wet or poo diaper if she is tired. Babies at this age manage to sleep for long periods with very full diapers, and they don't complain. When she wakes she would rather feed than have her diaper changed first.

HOW LONG CAN YOU LET A BABY CRY?

You can let a baby cry for as long as you can cope with it.

HOW TO COPE WITH THE CRYING

• BREATHE! When a baby is crying we tend to become anxious and hold our breath, even if she is not our baby. Babies are very intuitive little people, and they pick up on our anxiety and become even more agitated and anxious themselves. (Watch this happen in a room of adults with one crying baby!) Now take another deep breath and let it out very slowly. Allow your shoulders to drop from up around your earlobes, and let your belly and butt flop.

• Have your own learning experience with baby's crying in the morning. It is easier to cope with an uncomfortable situation

when the sun is up and we are fresh from
a night's sleep.

- Instead of looking at the clock, set yourself a chore to do, such as the washing up,
  having a shower, putting clothes out to dry,
  and so on, before responding to her. Listen
  to baby's crying and you will notice that a
  baby's crying is like waves in the sea—one
  minute, full and out of control, the next,
  more calm and in control. If you think that
  she is in control, then maybe hold back on
  stepping in to take over. Support her in
  learning to put herself to sleep.

Second and subsequent babies cry and learn to put
themselves to sleep simply because their parents are
busy with the toddler's needs and cannot respond immediately to the new baby's crying. Think of all your
friends who are second and third or fourth children
in their family, and they will appear just as "together"
and undamaged as their firstborn sibling.

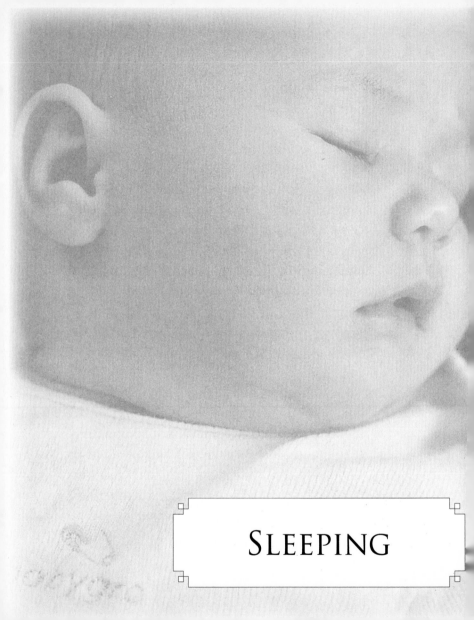

SLEEPING

For a new baby, "going to sleep" without any help is a skill he needs to learn. Some babies learn more quickly than others do, and a baby may take up to three months to achieve this.

If a baby is overtired and overhandled, then it takes him a lot longer to get to sleep and he will do a lot of crying.

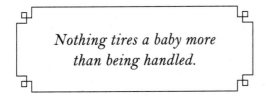

Nothing tires a baby more than being handled.

HOW MUCH SLEEP DOES A BABY NEED?

- On average, a newborn baby will sleep about 16½ hours in a 24-hour day. This is broken into 4 "day sleeps" and longer sleeps over an 8½-hour period at night.

If a baby is having 6–7 feedings in the 24 hours, and the feeding process takes about an hour with a diaper change, giving the feed, burping, wrapping, and back to bed, it can be seen that 6–7 hours have gone in "baby activity." This is about as much "up" time as baby can manage for the first few weeks.

- By 4 weeks of age, baby will sleep, on average, 15½ hours in the 24-hour day, with 3 longer day sleep periods and longer sleeps over a 9-hour period at night.

By now the feed times will be reducing a little, and you will have a handle on bathing, changing, and general "doing" for the baby. Baby will become more sociable—he may even be smiling occasionally. Now you can enjoy a little more "up" time with him, even though he still does not need playtime or entertainment.

- At 3 months of age, baby will sleep an average of 15 hours in a 24-hour period, with 3 shorter day sleeps and a longer nighttime sleep period of 7–10 hours.

Now we're talking good times! Baby might even be

sleeping through from his last feeding in the evening, say 9:00 or 10:00 p.m. to his early morning feed at 5:00 or 6:00 a.m. He will be content to have playtime, and there will even be lovely times of "talking" together.

One definition of sleep is dormancy or inactivity. Sometimes a "quietly sleeping baby" can in fact be resting in his bed quite peacefully with his eyes wide open. This quiet time that he is having with himself can also be regarded as his sleep time. Some babies have quite a lot of "quiet time"—aren't they lucky!

BABY'S SLEEP PATTERN

If baby is put to bed while still awake, he will learn to put himself to sleep.

This is fairly difficult to do in the beginning because he hasn't yet learned the skill. Most times he needs some sort of aid or comfort to help him get to sleep, such as patting, rocking, nursing, the bottle, the stroller, the car, the pacifier, holding, and so on.

The trouble with all of this is that baby will generally only stay asleep for about 20–30 minutes and the whole process has to be repeated. This is very exhausting for you, particularly if you have stairs or you are trying to get some sleep yourself!

It is also exhausting for baby as he has to keep calling out to you to come and help him get back to sleep. Understanding his sleep pattern will help you to understand why he does this.

Our sleeping state consists of many cycles of two different types of sleep, light or REM (rapid eye movement) sleep and deep sleep. A new baby has a sleep cycle that lasts for about 50 minutes, during which time he spends half his sleep time in light sleep and the other half in deep sleep. There will be two to three sleep cycles while he is asleep as the simple illustration shows on the following page.

Now let's look at what happens when baby has an aid to go to sleep and why he will only stay asleep for a short time. I will use the example of the breast as an aid.

When baby goes to the breast, his eyes are open

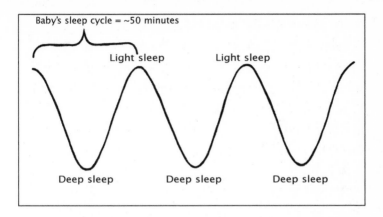

Baby's sleep cycle = ~50 minutes

Light sleep   Light sleep

Deep sleep   Deep sleep   Deep sleep

and he feeds heartily. Gradually, his eyes will close, and he will have a little munch time, then a rest, then another munch time, then a rest, and so on. He is actually in light sleep when he is doing this until he eventually passes into deep sleep and slips away from the breast. So we put him into bed, and twenty to thirty minutes later he is awake and calling out to us.

This is because he has reached the next light phase of his sleep cycle. If the aid that helped him to go to sleep in the beginning is no longer there (in this case, the breast), he will wake himself up looking for it so that he can get into deep sleep again.

SLEEP DEVELOPMENT

When a term baby is newly born, his sleeping pattern starts in the light-sleep stage, which is why he finds "going to sleep and staying asleep" difficult. This gradually changes over the first 100 days, when at about 3 months of age he will start his sleep in the deep-sleep stage, a pattern he will maintain throughout his life.

Supporting baby in learning to put himself to sleep in this period may provide a good foundation for him to become a "good sleeper" in the future.

SLEEPING POSITION

Sleeping on the back is the preferred option for newborn babies. If you choose to sleep your baby on the side, make sure that his lower arm or shoulder is well forward to prevent baby from rolling onto his tummy during sleep (SIDS Council of Australia directive, 2000).

If you choose to sleep your baby on his back, it is advisable to alternate the side his head falls to. This can be achieved by turning his head either to the right or left and then slightly turning his pelvis (hips) to face the same direction. This will help prevent a preference of head direction and the development of tight muscles in his neck and a slightly out of shape head. Of course baby will move his head around, particularly as he grows stronger, but at least start him sleeping with his head position alternating.

NOISES IN THE NIGHT

Babies are incredibly noisy creatures and not only when they are awake. You have probably discovered that your baby is very noisy when he is sleeping, particularly if, at night, he sleeps in the same room as you do. Don't be alarmed. Try to sleep through all the grunts, farts, squirms, and dreams.

An alternative is to move him into his own room to sleep.

SLEEPING ENVIRONMENT

Many first new babies spend a lot of time in a room where the curtains are drawn and there is no background noise. If he is having the occasional bad day, then this may be a good idea, but to live in this situation every day does not help him to grow up to be a versatile little person in a happening, noisy world. It also means that the family will have to stay home to provide this type of environment all the time. This does not seem like much fun.

A baby hears his first sounds while in the womb, so household noise is familiar to him and may even be comforting. Second and subsequent babies grow up with all sorts of toddler bangs and crashes going on around them and seem to be able to sleep through them.

Most babies learn to sleep through car and traffic noise and in the daylight while they are on an outing. If it is possible for you to let your baby sleep in a light environment with background family noise, then it will serve him and you in the long run.

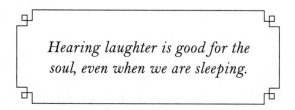

Hearing laughter is good for the soul, even when we are sleeping.

FEEDING

A great concern for a new parent is whether baby is getting enough to eat—how often, how much, and how.

HOW OFTEN SHOULD YOU FEED?

Generally, a newborn baby will feed 6–8 times in 24 hours. Occasionally a baby will thrive on only 5 feedings in 24 hours.

A daytime feeding routine can teach baby the concept of night and day if she is encouraged to feed every 3–4 hours during your daytime hours—that is, from the time that you get up in the morning to when you go to bed at night.

If baby has a long sleep in the day, then she will want to catch up on her feedings at night—this is not ideal!

If baby is demanding to be fed more often than every 3 hours, with sometimes up to 12 feedings in a 24-hour period, it is usually the result of her using the feedings as an aid to go to sleep. Try to extend the time between feedings to at least 3 hours, with that timing being from the beginning of a feeding to the beginning of the next feeding.

To enable baby and the breast to adjust, do this over a period of 1–3 days. On the first day extend the time between feedings by 10 minutes, the next day by 15–20 minutes, and continue in small steps until you reach the 3-hour limit.

Record on paper the times of the feedings, and you will be encouraged when you see the number of feedings in the 24 hours reducing to your goal of 6–8 feedings. There is no need to record feed times once you have reached this goal.

If baby demands it, the occasional day of 2-hourly breastfeedings may be necessary to boost a tired and depleted milk supply in order to meet her needs. On these days, reflect on how much rest and good food you are allowing yourself.

THE NIGHT FEEDING

If you keep baby's feedings regular in the daytime and let her call the shots at night, she will probably feed only once before 5:00 a.m.

This feeding may be a short sleepy feeding with NO diaper change unless absolutely necessary, if a disposable diaper is used overnight. By about 8 weeks of age, the feeding time can be completed in 12 minutes from the time you get out of bed to when you get back in.

You may be blessed with no night feeding by 10–12 weeks. Bliss!

Some babies regard "nighttime" as the period from their 6:00 p.m. feeding to their 1:00 or 2:00 a.m. feeding.

Waking baby for a 10:00 p.m. feeding makes no difference—she will still insist on a 2:00 a.m. feed. This is a bit of a nuisance having to wake from your sleep to feed her, but some parents find that this pattern (that is, skipping the 10:00 p.m. feeding) gives them the freedom to have a social life in the evening!

When baby starts "solids" at 4 months, she will drop the 2:00 a.m. feed and sleep from 6:00 or 7:00 p.m. to 4:00 or 5:00 a.m.

LENGTH OF A FEEDING

During the first 2–3 weeks, a baby's feeding time (which includes approximately 30–40 minutes at breast or bottle, a diaper change, and putting her back to her bed) will be about 60 minutes. If it takes longer than this, then look at where the extra time is going.

Gradually, this feed time will decrease until about 12 weeks, when the actual time taking milk may be between 5–10 minutes. Bliss!

FALLING ASLEEP BEFORE COMPLETING A FEEDING

In the first few weeks, a baby will often fall asleep before completing a feeding. This can be overcome by changing baby's diaper halfway through, rather than before, the feeding. Babies generally become quite alert when they have a diaper change and are quite willing to return to their feeding after it.

HOW MUCH?

The food for new babies for the first 4 months is either breast milk or formula milk. Quantities vary from baby to baby, with some babies needing large amounts and some babies thriving on less than the recommended guidelines.

If baby is gaining weight at a rate of about ⅓ pound a week or having at least 6 good wet or poo diapers each day, then she is feeding well.

Some babies may only gain about ⅕ pound one week and about ½ pound the next, but they average out at ⅓ pound, so don't be alarmed if this is happening. Look more at how content she is and how she is developing. Often babies follow the same growth patterns of their parents and their siblings when they were babies, so check with your families. It is difficult when confronted with a set of scales to remember that your baby is an individual and will grow at her own rate. Check with your doctor or baby health nurse if you are worried.

By 2 weeks of age, she needs to be offered both breasts at each feed. This does not mean that she will drink from the second breast each feed, but at least offer her the opportunity. The feed time will still be 30–40 minutes, with 25–30 minutes at the first breast and 5–10 minutes at the second breast. These feed times will reduce over the next 6–8 weeks.

If you are concerned about how much your baby is getting from the breast, always look at what comes out of her. What goes in (fluid or input) comes out (pee/poo or output).

This can be difficult to assess with disposable diapers, particularly when they are designed to last 12 hours. As an experiment, fill a measuring cup or bottle with up to 7 ounces of water. Pouring 1½ ounces at a time onto an unused diaper, judge the weight of it. Baby will often pee while having a diaper change or a bath, so count that as well. What goes in, must come out!

POSITION DURING FEEDING

When baby is feeding, check that she is comfortable so that the feeding is efficient and not tiring for her.

Whether she feeds from the bottle or the breast, check that her head is aligned with her body. This is more easily understood if we think of it in terms of facing straight ahead. To illustrate why this is important for her and her ability to have a comfortable feeding, experience this yourself. Facing straight ahead, take a swallow. Now turn your head so that it faces toward your shoulder and take another swallow. This is not a comfortable feeling. If baby is having this experience, she will soon start to fuss and will not feed properly.

Always check that a new baby has her head, shoulders, and hips facing the same direction when feeding. If breastfeeding, make sure her hips are tucked close to and facing toward your body.

BURPING

The idea that baby needs to have a burp after every feeding can lead to an event that leaves her thoroughly overhandled and tired, and the burper in a state of anxiety.

If there is no burp after 40–60 seconds, then carry on with the feeding or other baby needs. An effective way of "getting that burp" is

1. Position baby upright on your lap, with your hands gently supporting her chest, underarms, and neck.

2. Lift her gently until her bottom is no longer supported on your lap—in other words, she is now suspended with her body stretched out, rather than scrunched in a ball.

3. Kiss her forehead and head. This is very important, because when we kiss a baby, it is so delicious, not only for the kisser but also for the kissee, that you and baby relax. When the body relaxes, everything, including the tummy, gets a chance to work properly. If the body is not in a ball (or a "knot"), it can function better. If you are unable to kiss her, then rest your cheek against her and relax yourself by letting out your breath.

If you don't get that burp now, she'll give it to you later, either spontaneously as a burp, or with great gusto out the other end!

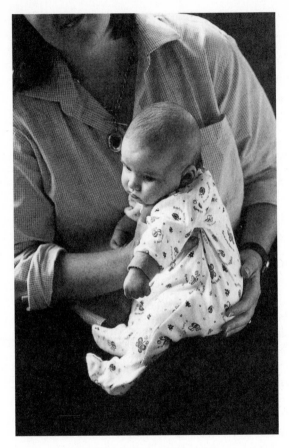

Position baby upright on lap.

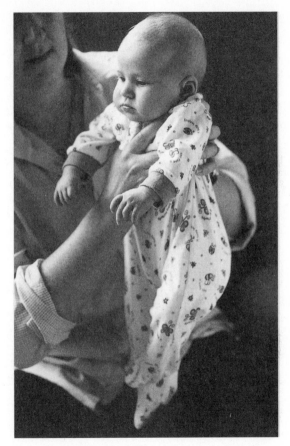

Lift baby until bottom is no longer supported.

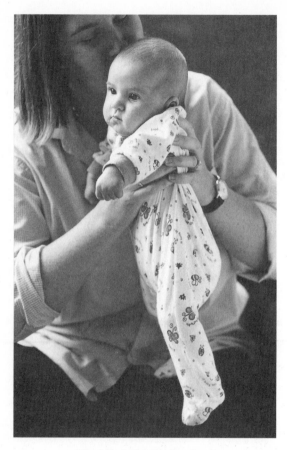

Kiss baby's forehead or head.

VOMITING

Sometime in the first few weeks, a newborn baby will probably have a very large and dramatic vomit. This can be quite alarming for the person who's in the firing line. It often requires a complete change of clothing for baby and probably you, with restorative washing of the couch and carpet. It looks like the whole feeding has come up.

When baby gives you back the occasional feeding, then it's because she is "full as a goog," or needs to get rid of mucous in her stomach. She does NOT need another feed immediately. Change her and put her to bed, and she will probably have a very good sleep, though she may wake a little earlier than usual for her next feed.

If baby is having lots of these big vomits and is not gaining weight, then you need to consult her doctor.

Some babies have little vomits or possets (the equivalent of one, two, or three teaspoons) after a feed, and continue to gain weight. This can happen throughout her first year and usually bothers you and the washing machine more than it does her. If you are concerned about this, then seek out your health professional for reassurance.

Occasionally a baby can appear distressed with vomiting (that is, she may be squirming, unsettled, and crying). This behavior needs to be checked out by her doctor.

HICCUPS

Most babies seem quite comfortable with hiccups. In fact, it is a familiar occurrence for them. Babies have their first hiccups in the womb, so when they have them after they are born, they can feel quite comforted.

Very rarely will a baby cry when hiccupping. She will often lie quite peacefully in her bed and hiccup her way to sleep.

Hiccups occur more frequently in newborn babies because their nervous and digestive systems are still developing after birth. They are not a frequent occurrence after baby has completed her unsettled behavior at around 9 weeks of age.

Hiccups are rhythmic. Babies love rhythm—such as patting, rocking, the car, and the sounds of the washing machine, dishwasher, and the vacuum cleaner. Baby's hiccups are her own rhythm, so let her have them when they occur!

COLIC

"Colic" is a term that is sometimes used by health professionals and grandmas to describe the very unsettled behavior of a baby.

Colic occurs when a baby gets tired and uptight. When we are tired, we forget to breathe deeply, the diaphragm gets tight, and the tummy tenses up and doesn't function easily. When baby begins to tire, she will cry, tighten up her tummy, and draw up her legs in an effort to get herself "back into the womb," where she felt comfortable and able to sleep.

The tummy discomfort of colic probably occurs because of tiredness rather than feeding.

"FUSSING" WHILE FEEDING

When a baby reaches 5–6 weeks of age, she may start "fussing" while she is feeding, particularly if she is feeding at the breast. This is because there is something she is not happy about, such as:

- A burp needs to come up.

  This will take about 45 seconds to relieve.

- The breast is too fast.

  Allow the breast to relieve itself by dripping for 40 seconds or so.

- The breast is too full, and baby has fed for as long as she needs to.

  A baby has her own inner wisdom, and she often knows when she has "had enough." If she continues to have wet diapers, is content, and thrives, then the breast supply will adjust itself.

  Also, be aware of how we, as adults, feed. Some meals are smaller than others.

- The breast is "empty."

Baby is becoming more efficient at feeding and doesn't need to be at the breast as long. If she is having a good output (wet/poo diapers), is contented between feedings, and is thriving, then the breast is producing enough milk.

If baby is demanding more feedings than usual, then the supply may be "down," but the extra 1–2 feedings a day will stimulate the breast to produce more. The breast operates on a principle of supply and demand.

If baby is formula fed, and she consistently empties each bottle, then add another 1–1½ ounces to each bottle.

Fussing while feeding occurs again when baby is around 8 weeks and 12 weeks of age. Be reassured by her output, her contentedness, and her continuing growth.

DEALING WITH THE FUSSING

As soon as baby starts to "fuss" when feeding (for

example, pulling her head back or side to side, or general squirming or agitation), stop the feeding and "burp" her for about 30 seconds. Continue the feeding on the second breast until she fusses. Then return her to the first breast until she fusses, which is when the feeding is over.

Observe how wet her diapers are for reassurance that she and the breast are just speeding up.

If baby is bottle-fed, then the process is the same, but the reasons are slightly different. Baby may need burping, the teat may be blocked, or she has just "had enough" for this meal, thank you!

THE BACK-TO-WORK BOTTLE

If a breastfeeding mother plans to return to work, or if she needs to have freedom from being available for a breastfeeding at some time in the future, then baby needs to have a bottle feeding of expressed milk or formula 2–3 times every week from the age of 6 weeks or earlier.

This is because most babies will refuse a bottle unless it is introduced into their routine at an early age.

There is no reason why a working mother would not be able to continue to breastfeed when she is with her baby and for the baby to have expressed breast milk or formula from a bottle when she isn't.

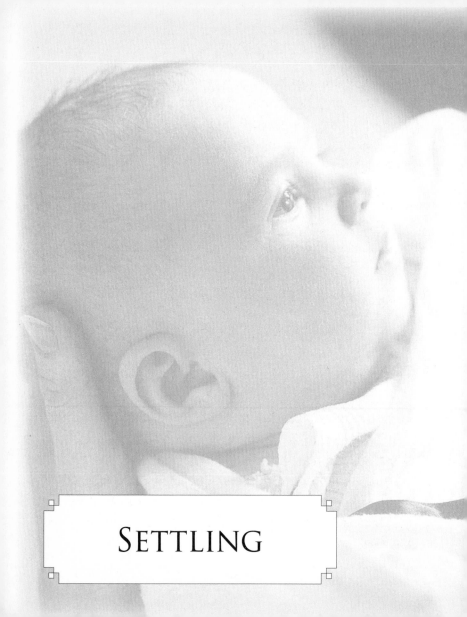

SETTLING

Settling the unsettled baby can be a time-consuming, tiring, frustrating experience, not only for the one who is trying to settle baby, but also for the baby.

As we explored in chapter 3, we found that crying is a natural event for a new baby, but even knowing this, having a crying baby can still be a very stressful time for new parents. This is because a baby's cry is so compelling that we have the urge to stop the crying and we can't always achieve it.

HOW LONG CAN YOU LET A BABY CRY?

You can let a baby cry for as long as you can cope with it. In the early days, this may only be for a very short time, but as time passes, coping becomes easier as confidence builds, and you become more familiar with the little person in your care.

The time to work on this confidence building is in the morning. Somehow, it is easier to cope with the baby crying when the sun is up, you are refreshed from sleep, and there are plenty of chores to be done.

Instead of taking too much notice of the clock,

make a pact with baby when you put him to bed that you will return to him if he needs you after you have washed your hair, or had your shower, or done the laundry, or switch the laundry to the dryer, or finished one of the other millions of things that need to be done.

Keeping the emphasis on whether he needs you is important, because *listening* to his cry is different to *hearing* his cry. When responding to a baby, pause to listen and determine whether he is in control. Is his cry winding down? Is he completely "losing it"? Is he just grizzling? Pause to listen and learn. Crying is his experience. Hearing his crying is ours.

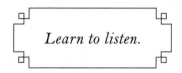

Learn to listen.

LISTEN BEFORE RESPONDING

When you pause to listen to baby's crying, take a very deep breath and let it out very slowly so that your shoulders relax, your tummy unwinds, and your buttock muscles drop. Then make your decision whether to respond to him or not.

If you make a decision to respond, here are some suggestions for helping him:

- Change his position in bed without lifting him from it. If you have him on his side, change sides. If he is on his back, adjust his head and pelvis position. (When we are sleeping or trying to go to sleep, we adjust our position until we feel comfortable. In other words, we toss and turn during sleep.)

- Use a pacifier.

- If he is lying on his side, place your hands on his body (shoulder and hip) and gently rock him a few times.

- Swaddle or wrap him securely.

THE PACIFIER

Every healthy term baby is born with a suck re-flex, along with about 30 other primitive reflexes such as the startle reflex, the step reflex, and the rooting reflex.

These reflexes start to disappear at about the time that the unsettled 2–9 week period disappears, and most term babies do not have them after 12–14 weeks of age.

Satisfying the suck reflex and the startle reflex is one way to help a newborn baby to settle.

The pacifier is a wonderful comfort for a baby who has a very strong suck reflex, and it avoids the use of the breast or bottle to satisfy his need to suck and suck and suck.

When first offering the pacifier, a baby may need some help in accepting it. A simple cherry shaped pacifier usually does the trick. If it is introduced just behind the top gum and directed toward the roof of his mouth, he will not gag and reject it. Allow him to suck or draw it into his mouth.

If he is very unsettled, calm him first with your

clean finger in the same way. When he has calmed, withdraw your finger and insert the pacifier.

Some babies will never accept a pacifier.

While a pacifier is an excellent comfort in the first 3 months, it is quite a good idea for baby to be weaned from the pacifier by about the age of 4 months.

The reason for this is that at about 7–8 months of age, it is quite normal for a baby to wake three or four times in a night, talk to the fairies, and then put himself back to sleep.

If baby needs a pacifier to help him back to sleep, and is unable to find it in the night, guess who has to. That's right. YOU—and you will need to do it three or four times every night!

This results in very tired, resentful, and cranky mommies and daddies and very tired and cranky babies.

SWADDLING (WRAPPING)

A baby spends 9 months in the womb—a warm and cozy environment, rocked with the mother's movements, and lulled by the rhythm of her heart-beat.

Toward the end of pregnancy, life in the womb is beginning to get a bit squished, so most babies wrap themselves in a ball, with their chin on their chest, their arms crossed in front of them, and their knees and legs tucked up toward their tummy. This is the fetal position.

When a newborn baby is not in this position, he can feel very uncomfortable and not nurtured, so when swaddling a baby to settle, try to create the fetal position for him. Here is one method of swaddling:

1. Use a soft, light wrap, baby blanket, or bassinette sheet (in summer, a muslin wrap is ideal). If rectangular in shape, fold over a good 8 inches of one long side. If the wrap is a more square shape, fold over a generous corner to reach toward the center of the wrap.

2. Place the base of baby's head on the fold line and tuck one of his arms well into the fold. Then tuck that end of the fold securely around his waist so that his arm is folded across his chest. Repeat this with his other arm.

3. Now lift baby up and hold him head up against your chest. Encourage his head to fold toward his chest, at the same time tucking his folded legs toward his tummy. BREATHE.

4. Place baby in his bed, preferably with his legs propped in the fetal position either against the end of his crib or bassinet, or bolstered with a folded towel.

This method of swaddling allows baby some movement of his arms without being disturbed by the startle (Moro) reflex, as well as freedom of his chest. If baby can move his arms, it encourages his breathing.

The occasional baby appears to struggle against his wrap, probably because he is very, very tired. If he is a baby who can settle with his hands free and not scratch or damage himself, then swaddle him as he likes it.

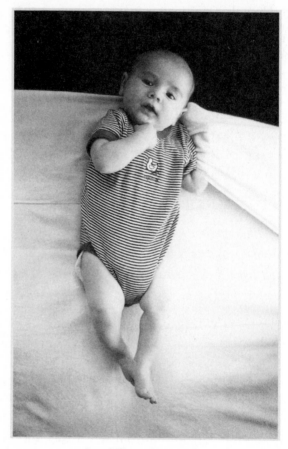

Swaddling steps 1 and 2.

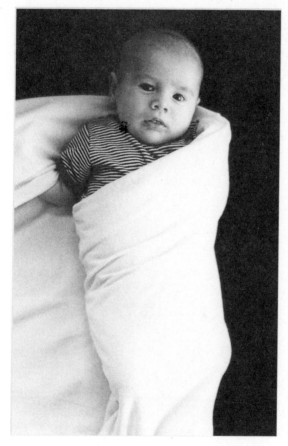

Swaddling step 2.

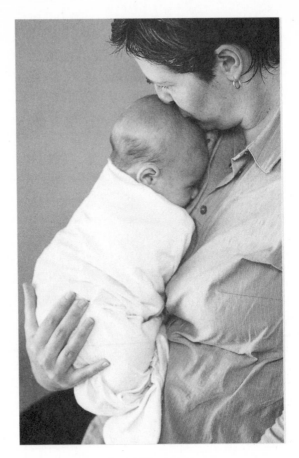

Swaddling step 3.

THE BATH

Another luxury of the womb is the relaxing warm fluid that baby bathes in. If you have tried to settle baby without success, then a warm bath may do the trick, particularly if he has recently been fed. A baby is more able to enjoy his bath if he has food in his tummy.

When he is undressed for the bath, massage baby with your warm hands, starting with his feet and working up his body using downward strokes. This can be very pleasurable for a baby, particularly if he is on his tummy and his chest and heart is "protected" by the surface on which he is lying. This position also allows for "tummy time," when he can lift his head and strengthen the muscles at the back of his neck.

If he feels vulnerable in the bath, place a warm wet washcloth across his chest and heart. This helps to keep him warm and gives him a feeling of "protection," and he may even "hang on" to it with his hands.

Dads are particularly good at massaging and bathing a baby. It is a wonderful way for a father to help and a great opportunity for him and his baby to spend quality time alone together. (See chapter 8—Having Fun.)

THE POUCH

Placing baby in a pouch close to your chest can be a wonderful comfort for an unsettled baby. It also is a very good time to take a walk and for you to get some exercise. As baby generally has his unsettled period during the evening when you are preparing or eating your meal, placing baby in a pouch means that you have your hands free to feed and nurture yourself. Dads are also particularly good at pouch time.

THE VERY, VERY UNSETTLED BABY

Some healthy babies seem to be incredibly unsettled in their first 100 days. For no obvious reason, they seem to cry louder and longer than other babies do. Their families need a lot of relief, support, and nurturing from relatives, friends, neighbors, and health professionals to help them through the first 6 months.

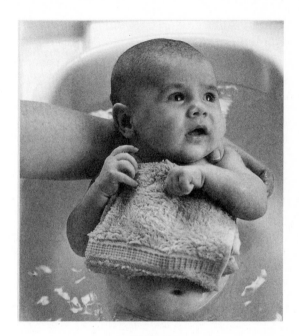

The bath.

If the crying continues, a complete medical check-up of baby with your family doctor or pediatrician is necessary.

Complementary therapies, such as cranio-sacral therapy or naturopathy with accredited practitioners can often help.

Take heart, for these little babies usually develop into the most delightful and happy little people.

HEART CHAKRA

In Eastern philosophy, there is a belief that an energy flows from the anus to the top of the head. This energy or "life force" has seven main vortexes, each one called a "chakra" or energy wheel, and is viewed as a consciousness center. It is believed that each chakra is concerned with very specific aspects of human behavior and development.

The Heart Chakra is the one with which we are most in touch and the one that we most want to protect. Whenever we receive bad news, our hand intuitively covers our heart in a protective movement. And, of course, when we are "in love," our "heart" feels wonderful. A new baby always tries to protect his Heart Chakra.

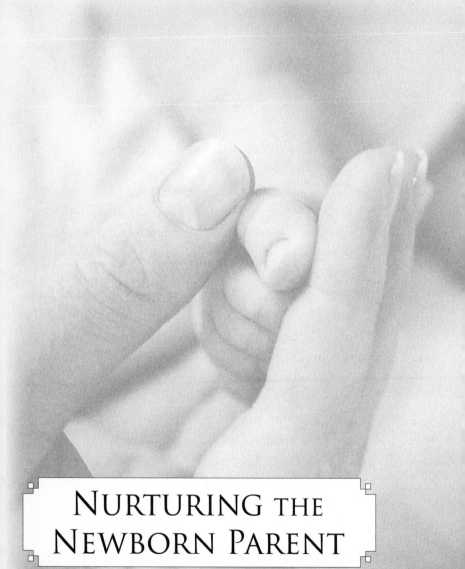

NURTURING THE NEWBORN PARENT

THE "BIRTHING" PROCESS

"Úrsula was barely over her forty days rest when the gypsies returned."

—Gabriel García Márquez,
One Hundred Years of Solitude

The "birthing" process only begins with the birth of a baby but it does not end until six weeks later. This has been forgotten in our Western culture.

Many other cultures, such as Greek and Asian, still acknowledge these six weeks as a very special time not only for the newborn baby but also particularly for the woman who has just given birth.

For women of the Victorian era it was known as the "lying in" period, when the newly delivered woman was constrained to remain in the home to rest and heal, and to be nurtured by the women of her family or community.

Now, a woman in today's society is allowed only a matter of hours of resting and healing, before "the gypsies" arrive to view the newborn baby, have a cup of tea, or even a baked dinner (prepared by the new-born mother, of course!). The gypsies then drift off into the night, leaving an exhausted, weeping mommy and baby.

Newborn daddies are generally very confused by now—wondering what is happening to this superwoman, who worked (maybe even ran the corporation) up until the moment of birth, held cordon bleu dinner parties, and managed the house.

What is happening to us as a couple?

When a baby comes into your life, you experience a miracle.

There are many life adjustments to realize. Suddenly, your social life is totally disrupted, and there is a tremendous feeling of new responsibility with a recognition that it will be like this for a long time.

There is exhaustion. There is a 24-hour daily commitment of nurturing, learning, coping, and growing. There is broken sleep. Sometimes it may feel like there is no sleep.

Be gentle with yourselves.

Remember, in wartime, sleep deprivation is used as a means of torture.

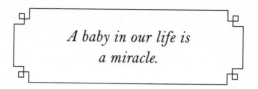

A baby in our life is a miracle.

There is so much to learn—about the baby, about yourself, about your partner, about your own parents, and about being a parent, as well as how to do things such as feeding, changing, using car seats, harnessing, folding the stroller, bathing baby, and so on.

Just going shopping with a 9-pound bundle is a major operation. In fact, sometimes it takes two adults, one stroller, one car, one grandma, two feedings, one diaper bag, your handbag, five breastpads, the car keys, and another feeding and diaper change just to get out of the house. And if that is all, then you are doing well!

Be gentle with yourselves.

You are learning, and in the beginning, things take a little bit longer than you would like.

"And it came to pass at the end of forty days, that Noah opened the window of the ark which he had made: . . . And he stayed yet other seven days; and again he sent forth the dove out of the ark; and the dove came in to him in the evening; and lo, in her mouth was an olive leaf pluckt off: so Noah knew that the waters were abated from off the earth."
—Genesis 8: 6–11

There is crying—let it happen. How lucky we are, as humans, to have tears that wash and release us.

In the forty days, the body lets go. It leaks. The womb releases the baby, the afterbirth, and its juices. The breasts let go and "leak." Our emotions let go and our eyes weep.

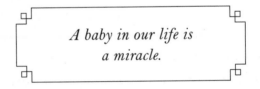

A baby in our life is a miracle.

Gradually this process lessens and completes by 5–6 weeks, and new strength comes.

Be gentle with yourselves.

This is a necessary event. Genesis is the birth.

The waters assuage, the ark resteth on Ararat, and Noah goes forth.

FEELINGS

Occasionally, some very uncomfortable feelings rise up in newborn parents. When you have done absolutely everything to settle a baby and she is still crying, then often feelings of resentment, or feelings of failure, or the feeling that you are "losing it" can happen.

This is a time to acknowledge those feelings and to remove yourself from the baby. Remind yourself that you are human; reach out to someone and let him or her know how you are feeling.

If there is no one there for you at a time of extreme feeling within you, place baby in her bed where she is quite safe and walk outside your home.

Walk to the mailbox, to the front gate, or even to the corner of the street. Baby is safe in her bed.

Reach out to anyone, even someone you don't know, and tell him or her how you are feeling.

This is not a part of parenting that is easily forgotten, and chances are that whoever you reach out to will remember only too well.

We are all human. Remind yourself that you are human.

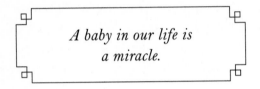

*A baby in our life is
a miracle.*

IT IS **NOT OKAY** TO ALLOW OUR ANGER AND
FRUSTRATION TO HARM THE BABY.

HAVING FUN

GETTING THINGS DONE

"Can any bus service rival the fine Hanley to Bagnall route in Staffordshire? In 1976 it was reported that the buses no longer stopped for passengers. This came to light when one of them, Mr. Bill Hancock, complained that buses on the outward journey regularly sailed past queues of up to thirty people.

"Councillor Arthur Cholerton then made transport history by stating that if these buses stopped to pick up passengers they would disrupt the time-table."

—Stephen Pile, *The Book of Heroic Failures: The Official Handbook of the Not Terribly Good Club*

There may be many, many times when you might think that you are a very good member of the "not terribly good club."

Well, the membership is huge, so search out some of the other members and have a good laugh. Some of them probably live next door and you never knew it!

Many of the funniest books written are drawn on memories of family bumblings. Are they really bumblings, or are these events just another way of doing things?

Consider a 12-minute diaper change where the whole time is taken up in trying to work out if the picture goes to the back or the front or the side. For those who know that the picture goes to the front of a disposable diaper, then the whole event can be staged in about 1–2 minutes. If you don't know, then it can take up to 12 minutes and even then the picture may not end up at the front, but the diaper will be on, baby dry, and the person who changed the diaper fairly proud of it all.

Now the purpose of this message is to point out that there are many ways of doing things, and it doesn't always have to be my way.

If it does, then there will not be a lot of fun all round.

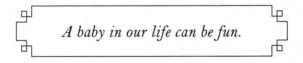

A baby in our life can be fun.

We all have our own unique beliefs and our own ways of doing things—baby doesn't really care, so long as the person "doing" is relaxed and loving. Sometimes parents or caregivers can feel overwhelmed when someone hovers over them telling them how to do things with the baby, and they then end up not enjoying handling the baby.

This can result in couples snapping at each other, particularly when they are very tired and feeling tense. This tension also affects the baby's behavior. Did you know that research has revealed that there are over 250 different ways of washing the dishes? Does it really matter?

If there is to be fun all round, then love and laughter beats "perfection" any day!

PLAYTIME

A baby is not ready for playtime until he is smiling and beginning to "mouth" words. Smiling can start in the first week, but some babies might not smile until about 8 weeks of age. The average is 4–6 weeks, and when it happens, it is one of the most warming and wonderful moments.

When a term baby is about 1 week old, he is able

to see the blurry outline of his mother's face and features from the distance of her breast (about 10–12 inches). At 4 weeks, a baby will gaze at whoever is holding him, studying every part of that face. This is his learning and "up" time.

Within a few weeks, he will be content to lie quietly in his bed and gaze at a venetian blind or ceiling fan.

At the end of his first 100 days, he will regard his hands and focus on toys within 10 feet. His color vision is starting to develop, and he will recognize his parents when they come into the room. He will move his head to observe his surroundings.

A baby's attention span is a developing thing. Watch his behavior. If he "shuts down," he will stop smiling. He will yawn, become agitated, and eventually grizzle. He has had enough playtime.

A baby does not get bored. He gets tired.

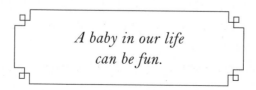

*A baby in our life
can be fun.*

HOLIDAYS, HOUSEGUESTS, AND ILLNESSES

When there is a change in routine, such as going on a vacation, having friends and relatives to stay, moving, or someone getting sick, a baby can lose the plot, and his behavior will regress to his previous stage of development. This is not permanent. He just needs time and support to get back on track, particularly with his sleeping and feeding patterns.

Parents can feel slightly shell-shocked with this regression and need patience and understanding.

Holidays, houseguests, and illnesses are part of our lives. Families need holidays and recreation, fun and laughter, and a change of place and pace.

The little illnesses along the way? Well, they are not so much fun, but they build immunity.

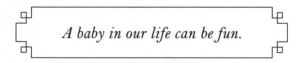

A baby in our life can be fun.

WHEN THERE IS NOT MUCH FUN

Many parents notice a happy and positive change in how they feel about their new life with a baby at about 5–6 weeks after the birth.

If a newborn parent still feels weepy, anxious, or "down" after this period, then it is time to talk about it with a health professional such as the family doctor.

There is no shame in feeling this way, but it does affect the "having fun" part of having a baby in your life.

There are many ways of being supported through these feelings, so that "falling in love" with your baby and with your life can happen sooner. Search for help and guidance. If you are not happy with what you hear, seek out another opinion.

Schedules are flexible—so stop for friends and family on the way and have fun. You are on the journey of your life.

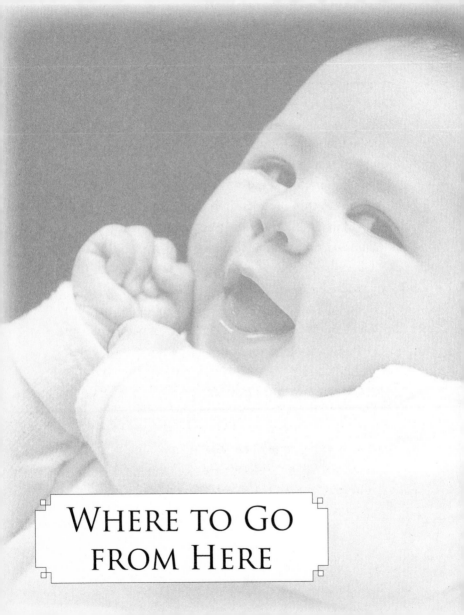

WHERE TO GO FROM HERE

At about 12 weeks of age a baby will settle and sleep a lot better if:

- She is not wrapped or swaddled. However, if it is a cue for sleep, then continue to wrap, but leave baby's hands free so that if she wants to comfort herself she can find her fingers or thumbs. Leaving baby's hands free also enables her to get herself out of trouble when she begins to move around her bed.

- She is put to sleep in a crib rather than a bassinet.

- There is a warm absorbent layer between the bottom sheet and the cold/hot covering of the mattress. Cotton blankets that you no longer use for swaddling or a bath towel or a mattress protector work well. This also protects the mattress from baby's spills and leaks.

- She is dressed and covered in layers. It is preferable to use a cotton singlet in the first 12 months, even if, on a very hot day, she is dressed in only her singlet and diaper. How many layers? One more layer than you have on is a good guide.

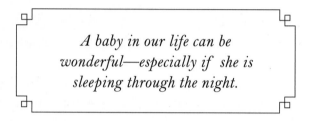

A baby in our life can be wonderful—especially if she is sleeping through the night.

On about the 100th day, the "sleeping through the night" bubble will probably burst!

Your breastfed baby is hungry, and she is getting ready to have solid food. But that all happens in the second 100 days, and that's another book!

ABOUT THE AUTHOR

Margaret Stephenson Meere, BA, BHSc, RN, RM, is an early childhood health practitioner based in Sydney.

A registered nurse and midwife with working experience in both Australia and the UK spanning nearly four decades, Margaret came to the realization in the 1980s that education and prevention, rather than treatment and cure, is preferable for a healthy life experience.

Margaret brings to her work a belief in holistic medicine, having trained in cranio-sacral therapy (pediatrics) with the Upledger Institute and also in Hellerwork postural correction and counseling. She studied human bioscience with a major in history to complete her bachelor of arts. Her work as an early childhood and family health nurse consultant commenced after she completed her Tresillian child and family health care training.

A mother of four sons and grandmother of five grandchildren, she spends most of her time on the mid north coast of New South Wales. Margaret's first book, *Baby's First 100 Days*, was first published in 2001. Her second book, *The Child Within the Lotus*, was published in 2009.